Sex, the Heart and Er

*To Emma Martin, Elaine McGing
and Alethea Cooper for endless support*

Sex, the Heart and Erectile Dysfunction

Graham Jackson FRCP FESC FACC

Consultant Cardiologist

Guy's and St Thomas' Hospital Trust

London

UK

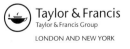

Taylor & Francis
Taylor & Francis Group

LONDON AND NEW YORK

A MARTIN DUNITZ BOOK

© 2004 Taylor & Francis, an imprint of the Taylor & Francis Group

First published in the United Kingdom in 2004
by Taylor & Francis, an imprint of the Taylor & Francis Group, 11 New Fetter Lane, London
EC4P 4EE

Tel.:   +44 (0) 20 7583 9855
Fax.:   +44 (0) 20 7842 2298
E-mail: info@dunitz.co.uk
Website: http://www.dunitz.co.uk

Although every effort has been made to ensure that all owners of copyright material have
been acknowledged in this publication, we would be glad to acknowledge in subsequent
reprints or editions any omissions brought to our attention.

A CIP record for this book is available from the British Library.

Library of Congress Cataloging-in-Publication Data

Data available on application

ISBN 1-84184-256-7

Distributed in North and South America by

Taylor & Francis
2000 NW Corporate Blvd
Boca Raton, FL 33431, USA

Within Continental USA
Tel.: 800 272 7737; Fax.: 800 374 3401
Outside Continental USA
Tel.: 561 994 0555; Fax.: 561 361 6018
E-mail: orders@crcpress.com

Distributed in the rest of the world by
Thomson Publishing Services
Cheriton House
North Way
Andover, Hampshire SP10 5BE, UK
Tel.: +44 (0)1264 332424
E-mail: salesorder.tandf@thomsonpublishingservices.co.uk

Printed and bound in Italy by Printer Trento.

Contents

Preface

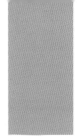

While there is more to life than sexual intercourse, sex is an important part of life and should be enjoyed throughout life. Cardiac patients are often afraid of having sex in the belief that it might precipitate a myocardial infarct or even lead to sudden death. This fear may be shared with their partners and also concern health care professionals. In addition, sexual dysfunction, usually male erectile dysfunction, is common in patients with vascular disease or in those at high risk for vascular disease and this in itself, because of the failure to address the problem, may compound sexual anxieties.

Sex, the Heart and Erectile Dysfunction focuses on the cardiovascular response to sex and specifically aims to address safety issues, advising patients and treating sexual dysfunction in cardiac patients. It is intended for health care professionals involved in the management of this group of patients. Many patients are reluctant to discuss sex and I hope this Pocketbook will encourage doctors, nurses and all involved with the management of cardiac patients to initiate discussion.

While sex is a serious subject, it is also full of humour and it is important not to be afraid of using humour to break the ice.

Graham Jackson

Sex and the heart – the physiological response

Sex between a couple in a long-standing relationship is not particularly stressful to the heart. In general, the physiological cost of sexual activity is similar to exercise of mild-to-moderate intensity for the average middle-aged person going about other aspects of normal daily life.[1]

Using ambulatory monitoring studies of heart rate and blood pressure, the following measurements have been determined:

- Average maximal heart rate during sex is 110–130 beats/min.
- Average peak systolic blood pressure is 150–180 mmHg.
- Average rate pressure product calculates at 16,000–23,000.

These levels are no greater than those observed for, say, walking, travelling to work or climbing stairs, and can be compared using METs (metabolic equivalent of the task). One MET is the relative energy demand for oxygen usage in the resting state and approximates to 3.5ml/kg body weight/minute.[2]

As shown in Table 1.1, the level of exertion associated with a range of daily activities can be compared with the cardiac demands of sex, providing a useful and simple guide. A useful outpatient baseline for advice is the 1 mile (1.5 km) in 20 minutes on the flat, perhaps supplemented by asking if the patient can briskly climb up and down two flights of stairs.

Casual sex with a relatively unfamiliar partner may increase the cardiac stress, particularly if there is an age mismatch. This may follow a meal and alcohol consumption, both of which will increase cardiac work. Although sex rarely causes a significant cardiac event, when it does happen, in 75% of cases the sex is casual and 90% of the people affected are men.

Table 1.1 MET equivalents

Daily activity	MET score rating
Sexual intercourse with established partner	
lower range ('normal')	2–3
lower range orgasm	3–4
upper range (vigorous activity)	5–6
Lifting and carrying objects (9–20 kg)	4–5
Walking one mile in 20 minutes on the level	3–4
Golf	4–5
Gardening (digging)	3–5
DIY, wallpapering, etc.	4–5
Light housework, e.g. ironing, polishing	2–4
Heavy housework, e.g. making beds, scrubbing floors, cleaning windows	3–6

The average duration of sex is 5–15 minutes, so sex is neither a severe cardiac stress nor a sustained cardiac stress.

Exercise testing

Where there are doubts about the safety of sex, an exercise ECG can be performed. Using METs, sex is equivalent to 3–4 minutes of the standard Bruce treadmill protocol. If the person can manage at least 4 minutes on the treadmill without significant symptoms, such as ECG evidence of ischaemia, a fall in systolic blood pressure or dangerous arrhythmias, it will be safe to advise on sexual activity. If the subject is unable to perform an exercise test because of mobility problems, a pharmacological stress test should be used (e.g. dobutamine stress echocardiography). If the partner is anxious, then by watching the stress test they can be reassured.

If 3–4 METs are not achieved, further evaluation by angiography is recommended.

Positions

As long as the couple are comfortable (not stressed) by the sexual position they use, there is no evidence of increased cardiac stress to the man or the woman. Man on top, woman on top, side to side or oral sex are equivalent. In homosexual male relationships (other than casual), anal intercourse is not associated with increased cardiac stress provided proper lubrication is used.

Key points
- Sex is not particularly stressful to the heart.
- Advice can be given by equating sex to other normal daily activities.
- If in doubt, an exercise test is recommended.

Sex and cardiac risk

Myocardial infarction

There is only a small degree of risk associated with sex. According to a US study the relative risk of a myocardial infarct (MI) during the 2 hours following sexual activity was:[3]

- All patients 2.5 (1.7–3.7)[*]
- Men 2.7 (1.8–4.0)
- Women 1.3 (0.3–5.2)
- Previous MI 2.9 (1.3–6.5)
- Sedentary life 3.0 (2.0–4.5)
- Physically active 1.2 (0.4–3.7)

The baseline absolute risk of an MI during normal daily life is low – one chance in a million per hour for a healthy adult and 10 chances in a million per hour for a patient with documented cardiac disease. Therefore, during the two hours post-sex, the risk increases to 2.5 in a million for a healthy adult and 25 in a million for a patient with documented cardiac disease; but, importantly, there is no risk increase in those who are physically active.

A similar study from Sweden has reported identical findings.[4] If we take a baseline annual rate of 1% for a 50-year-old man, as a result of weekly sexual activity, the risk of an MI increases to 1.01% in those without a history of a previous MI and to 1.1% in those with a previous history.

[*]Confidence limits in brackets

Key points

▓ The absolute risk of an MI during sex is very low.
▓ Absolute risk is reduced by regular physical activity – the physically fit will be sexually fit.

Death

Coital sudden death is very rare. In 3 large studies, sex activity-related death was 0.6% in Japan, 0.18% in Frankfurt and 1.7% in Berlin.[1] Extramarital sex was responsible for 75%, 75% and 77%, respectively, and the victims were men in 82%, 94% and 93% of cases, respectively. An older man with a younger woman was the commonest scenario – too much to eat, too much to drink and too much to prove.

Key points

▓ Death during sex is rare.
▓ Extramarital (casual) sex is more risky.

Erectile dysfunction: the problem

Erectile dysfunction (ED) is defined as the persistent inability to achieve and then maintain an erection to permit sexual intercourse.[5]

In the general population ED affects, to a varying severity, up to 52% of men aged 40–70 years. In 1995, it was estimated that ED affected over 152 million men worldwide. As ED increases in incidence with age (a man aged 70 years is three times more likely to have ED than a man of 40 years) and as we are an ageing population, it is estimated that by the year 2025, over 300 million men worldwide will suffer some degree of ED.[6]

Consequences

ED is a very distressing condition that not only has a negative impact on the man's sexual ability but also has damaging repercussions on the couple's quality of life. ED leads to depression, anxiety and loss of self-esteem and can contribute significantly to 20% of marital breakdowns.[7] Men are reluctant to seek help for fear of not being taken seriously or out of embarrassment (Figure 3.1) and become isolated within their relationship, which may lose all aspects of intimate contact.[8] The tragedy is that treatment is readily available and highly effective, yet for many not utilized. Nearly 90% of men who have successful treatment for their ED report significant improvement of emotional and overall well-being. Encouraging men alone or with their partners to seek help is therefore a major challenge.

Causes of ED

The aetiology of ED was regarded until recently to be predominantly psychogenic, but with our increasing knowledge of the physiology of penile

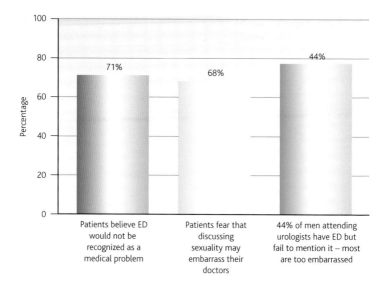

Figure 3.1 Patients reluctant to talk to their doctors about erectile dysfunction – why? (*Source*: Marwick C. *JAMA* 1999; **281**: 2173–4)

erection and pathophysiology of ED, it is now recognized to be mainly an organic condition, with vascular disease responsible for 70% of cases. For most men, the cause may be multifactoral, especially in the elderly (75% of men aged over 80 years have ED), with endocrine, cellular, neural and iatrogenic causes exacerbating vascular ED or being independently causative. Organic ED will have psychological consequences which must be recognized and addressed as part of the overall management.[2,9]

Physiology of penile erection

A penile erection occurs in response to stimuli which may be visual, erotic, olfactory, auditory and tactile.[10] It is a neurovascular event that may be modulated by hormonal and psychological factors. On sexual stimulation, there is increased parasympathetic activity and decreased sympathetic activity. The parasympathetic nerves release the neurotransmitters, the most important of which is nitric oxide (NO), which is also released by the endothelium (Figure 3.2). NO activates a soluble guanylate cyclase, which in turn raises the intracellular concentration of cyclic guanosine monophosphate (cGMP). Cyclic GMP then activates a specific protein kinase, which leads to the inhibition of calcium channels and the opening of potassium channels. The end result is relaxation of the smooth muscle in the penile arteries and the spongy tissue of the corpora cavernosa. A several-fold increase in blood flow to the penis occurs and, as the penis becomes erect with intracavernous pressures up to 100 mgHg, venous out-

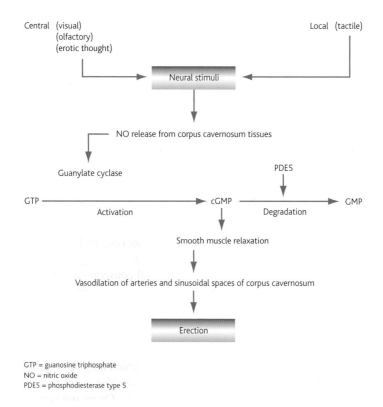

Figure 3.2 Role of PDE5 in penile erection. (*Source:* Giuliano F. *Eur Heart J Suppl.* 2002; **4**(suppl H): H7–H12)

flow is occluded and the erection is sustained. Cyclic GMP is regulated by phosphodiesterase type 5 (PDE5), which enzymatically degrades and inactivates this cyclic nucleotide. Penile rigidity is lost and flaccidity returns.

When we consider the cascade of events, there are several areas where disturbances in the neurovascular sequence might lead to ED, but most attention has focused on PDE5 and its inhibition.

Vasculogenic ED

Vascular disease is the most common cause of ED, with endothelial dysfunction being the common denominator. While atherosclerosis is the commonest vascular disease linked to ED, its risk factors are associated with the development of ED (Figure 3.3), and these include:

▥ Cigarette smoking
▥ Hypertension
▥ Hyperlipidaemia
▥ Diabetes

Before attributing the ED to a purely vascular cause, a detailed assessment of the patient's history may identify other factors that are contributory or occasionally the main reason why ED has developed.

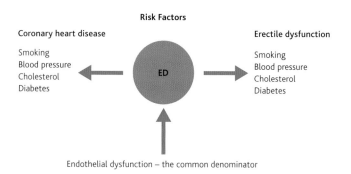

Figure 3.3 Risk factors. (*Source:* Solomon H *et al. Heart* 2003; **89**:251–4)

Psychogenic ED

The importance of sexual activity to the male psyche is paramount and all men with ED are affected by psychological issues which lead to general anxiety, depression and performance-related anxiety. The presence of normal nocturnal erections in men with ED identifies the neurovascular mechanisms as being intact and points to a predominantly psychogenic cause for ED (Table 3.1).

Table 3.1 *Differentiating organic and psychological ED*

Organic	Psychogenic
Onset is gradual	Sudden onset
Impaired or absent morning erections	Normal morning erections
Normal sexual history	Problems in sexual history
Normal sex drive (libido)	Relationship issues
Constant	Specific circumstance
Note: Organic and psychogenic causes often overlap – they are not mutually exclusive	

Psychosexual counselling is advised for those patients who may suffer stress at work or experience stressful personal or financial matters. There may be relationship issues, performance anxiety, depression, lack of sexual education or sexual problems with the partner.

Neurological ED

Both central and peripheral nervous diseases can lead to ED. Aside from obvious traumas, such as spinal cord injury, or a specific disease, such as multiple sclerosis, depression, Parkinson's disease and cerebrovascular disease can complicate both the assessment and management of vasculogenic ED.

Endocrine-induced ED

Testosterone is important for both male sex drive and penile erection. A reduction in libido may be a consequence of testicular male hypogonadism

– nocturnal erections may diminish and there may be less penile rigidity or difficulty in sustaining an erection. Serum testosterone measurements should be taken when loss of libido is a significant complaint. This can also occur in men with predominantly vasculogenic ED, as the age groups at presentation are similar.

Iatrogenic ED

A large number of drugs, whether prescribed or recreational, can affect sexual function (Table 3.2). The negative impact may be on erection, ejaculation or sex drive. There is little evidence that changing cardiovascular drug therapy will restore erectile function, suggesting it is the underlying disease process that is more important. However, if there is a strong temporal relationship between the commencement of pharmacological treatment and the onset of ED (2–4 weeks), it is logical to change therapy if it is safe to do so. Antihypertensive agents, especially thiazide diuretics, are the most frequently incriminated and a switch to angiotensin II receptor antagonists or alpha-blockers should be considered. Where drugs are prognostically important, such as beta-blockers post-infarction, the decision to discontinue therapy should be approached with caution and only undertaken after considering overall risks.[2]

Radical pelvic surgery may damage the parasympathetic nerves that run close to the prostate. Radiotherapy for bladder, prostate or rectal cancer can lead to ED secondary to vasculogenic damage, perhaps superimposed on surgical nerve damage.

Key points
- ED is common.
- ED has distressing consequences.
- ED is predominantly vascular.
- Psychosocial issues may coincide – a mixed aetiology.

Table 3.2 Drugs linked to ED

Cardiovascular drugs
Thiazide diuretics
Beta-blockers
Calcium antagonists
Centrally acting agents
methyldopa
clonidine, reserpine
ganglion blockers
Digoxin
Lipid-lowering agents
ACE inhibitors
Recreational drugs
Alcohol
Marijuana
Amphetamines
Cocaine
Anabolic steroids
Heroin
Psychotropic drugs
Major tranquillizers
Anxiolytics and hypnotics
Tricyclic antidepressants
Selective serotonin reuptake inhibitors
Endocrine drugs
Antiandrogens
Oestrogens
LHRH analogues
Testosterone

(cont)

Table 3.2 *Drugs linked to ED (cont)*

Others
Cimetidine and ranitidine
Metoclopramide
Carbamazepine

Erectile dysfunction and cardiovascular disease

Prevalence

The Massachusetts Male Agency Study (MMAS) was a random sample cross-sectional observation study of 1709 healthy men aged 40–70 years which assessed the impact of ageing on a wide range of health-related issues.[11] Fifty-two per cent of respondents reported some degree of ED (17% mild, 25% moderate, 10% complete) with prevalence increasing with age. Cardiovascular disease was significantly associated with ED. The incidence was doubled in hypertensives, tripled in diabetic patients, and quadrupled in patients with established coronary artery disease (CAD). Cigarette smoking increased the prevalence two-fold for all of these conditions, and a positive relationship was found for reduced HDL cholesterol and ED.

The association between hyperlipidaemia and ED has been studied in apparently healthy men who complained of ED.[9,12] Over 60% had hyperlipidaemia, and 90% of these men had evidence of penile arterial disease using Doppler ultrasound investigations. Diabetes is commonly associated with ED, with a prevalence of 50% (range: 27–70% depending on age and disease severity). The onset of ED usually occurs within the first 10 years of diagnosis.[13]

Men older than 50 years with established CAD have an ED incidence of 40%, and in those post-infarct or following vascular surgery, the incidence ranges from 39 to 64% depending on the diagnostic criteria.

The endothelial link

Endothelial dysfunction is defined as an abnormal endothelial response leading to a reduction in the bioavailability of NO and impaired vasodilation. This results in an inability of the smooth muscle cells to relax throughout the vasculature. The reduced bioavailability of NO leads to the development of atherosclerosis, increased platelet aggregation, vessel wall inflammation and smooth muscle cell proliferation. Endothelial dysfunction is therefore common to cardiovascular disease and ED, establishing an intimate link between the two pathologies, which explains to a significant degree the prevalence of ED in the conditions associated with endothelial dysfunction (e.g. diabetes) and the toxic risk factors such as cigarette smoking.[14]

ED as a marker of vascular disease

Since ED and vascular disease share the same risk factors, the possibility arises that ED in an otherwise asymptomatic man may be a marker of silent vascular disease, especially CAD. This has now been established to be the case and represents an important new means of identifying those at vascular risk.[15]

Pritzker studied 50 asymptomatic men (other than ED) aged 40–60 years who had cardiovascular risk factors (multiple risk factors in 80%).[16] Exercise electrocardiography was abnormal in 28 men and subsequent coronary angiography in 20 identified severe CAD in 6, moderate two-vessel disease in 7 and significant single-vessel CAD in a further 7. In a study of 132 men attending day care angiography, 65% had some degree of ED and more than 50% had experienced ED before their CAD diagnosis had been made.[17] ED also correlates with the severity of CAD, with single-vessel disease patients having less difficulty obtaining an erection (Figure 4.1).[18] In our own study of 178 men presenting with ED to a urology service, a high incidence of cardiovascular risk factors was noted with a significant number previously undetected or poorly controlled (Figure 4.2).[19]

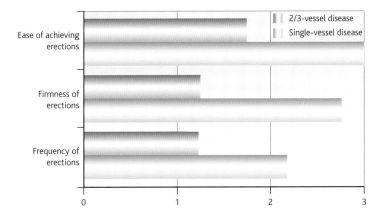

Figure 4.1 Degree of erectile dysfunction related to the extent of coronary artery disease (n=40). (*Source:* Adapted from Greenstein A *et al*. *Int J Impot Res* 1997; **9**: 123–6)

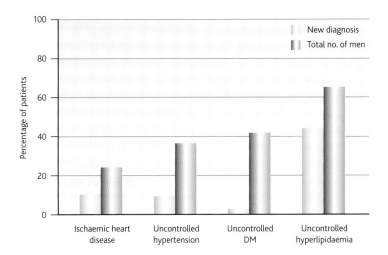

Figure 4.2 The prevalence of cardiovascular risk factors in a cohort of 178 men presenting with erectile dysfunction to a urology service. (*Source:* Solomon H *et al*. *Int J Impot Res* 2002; **14**: S74)

Key points

- ED is common in cardiac patients.
- ED in a man without cardiac symptoms may be a marker for silent vascular disease which should be screened for.
- ED can reflect poorly controlled vascular risk factors.
- Any asymptomatic man with ED without an obvious cause should be screened for vascular disease and have blood glucose, lipids and blood pressure measurements. Those at risk should undergo exercise electrocardiography.

Treating erectile dysfunction in cardiac patients

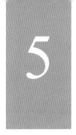

Guidelines

Recognizing the need for advice on management, two consensus panels (UK and US) have produced similar guidelines dividing risk into three practical categories with management recommendations.[2,20] The UK consensus guidelines have recently been updated (Table 5.1).[2] It is recommended that all men with ED should undergo a full medical assessment (Appendix 2). Baseline physical activity needs to be established and cardiovascular risk graded low, intermediate or high. Most patients with low or intermediate cardiac risk can have their ED managed in the outpatient or primary care setting.

Measurements of ED

As ED is a very personal problem, questionnaires have been developed for self-administration in the natural home (private) setting (Appendix 1). The most commonly used are the International Index of Erectile Function (IIEF), Sexual Encounter Profile (SEP) and Global Assessment Questionnaire (GAQ) (Table 5.2).[21] Using the IIEF scoring system with the questions relating to the previous 4 weeks, ED is classed as severe (scores 1–10), moderate (11–16), mild (17–25) and normal (26 and above). Therapeutic success can be monitored by repeating questionnaires at regular intervals and, of course, failure to respond will also become evident.

Treating ED in the cardiac patient

There is no evidence that treating ED in cardiac patients increases cardiac risk, with the proviso that the patient is properly assessed and the couple or

Table 5.1 Management algorithm according to graded risk

Grading or risk	Cardiovascular status upon presentation	ED management recommendations for the primary care physician
Low risk	• Controlled hypertension • Asymptomatic ≤3 risk factors for CAD – excluding age and gender • Mild valvular disease • Minimal/mild stable angina (Appendix 4) • Post successful revascularization • CHF (I) (Appendix 5)	• Manage within the primary care setting • Review treatment options with patient and his partner (where possible)
Intermediate risk	• Recent MI or CVA (i.e. within last 6 weeks) • LVD/CHF (II) (Appendix 5) • Murmur of unknown cause • Moderate stable angina (Appendix 4) • Heart transplant • Recurrent TIAs • Asymptomatic but >3 risk factors for CAD – ↔ excluding age and gender	• Specialised evaluation recommended (e.g. exercise test for angina, Echo for murmur) • Patient to be placed in high or low risk category, depending upon outcome of testing ED treatment can be initiated but exercise testing recommended to stratify risk

Table 5.1 Management algorithm according to graded risk (cont)

Grading or risk	Cardiovascular status upon presentation	ED management recommendations for the primary care physician
High risk	• Severe or unstable or refractory angina (Appendix 4) • Uncontrolled hypertension (SBP > 180 mmHg) • CHF (III, IV) (Appendix 5) • Recent MI or CVA (i.e. within last 14 days) • High risk arrhythmias • Hypertrophic cardiomyopathy • Moderate/severe valve disease	• Refer for specialized cardiac evaluation and management • Treatment for ED to be deferred until cardiac condition established and/or specialist evaluation completed

CAD, coronary artery disease; MI, myocardial infarction; CVA, cerebral vascular accident; CHF, congestive heart failure; LVD, left ventricular dysfunction; SBP, systolic blood pressure; ED, erectile dysfunction; TIA, transient ischaemic attack

Table 5.2 Erectile dysfunction assessment instruments

a)	IIEF erectile dysfunction domain score	Score range*
1.	Over the past four weeks, how often were you able to get an erection during sexual activity?	0–5
2.	Over the past four weeks, when you had erections with sexual stimulation, how often were your erections hard enough for penetration?	0–5
3.	Over the past four weeks, when you attempted sexual intercourse, how often were you able to penetrate (enter) your partner?	0–5
4.	Over the past four weeks, during sexual intercourse, how often were you able to maintain your erection after you had penetrated (entered) your partner?	0–5
5.	Over the past four weeks, during sexual intercourse, how difficult was it to maintain your erection to completion of intercourse	0–5
6.	Over the past four weeks, how do you rate your confidence that you can keep your erection?	1–5
	Total range	1–30*
b)	**Sexual encounter profile (SEP)**	
2.	Were you able to insert your penis into your partner's vagina?	Yes/No
3.	Did your erection last long enough to have successful intercourse	Yes/No
c)	**Global assessment questionnaire (GAQ)**	
1.	Has the treatment you have been taking improved your erections?	Yes/No

*The higher the score, the better is the erectile function

individual (self-stimulation may be the only form of sexual activity) are properly counselled.[2] There is more to sex than an erect penis and couples may, as a consequence of the presence of ED, have lost over time the touching, caring aspects of an intimate relationship. Detailed advice and support (short and long term) is an essential part of overall management. Oral drug therapy is the most widely used because of its acceptability and effectiveness, yet all therapies have a place in management. The philosophy is not to accept failure and to be positive during a time which for many men and their partners must be full of uncertainties and difficult.

Key points

- Guidelines have been established to facilitate management.
- The majority of cardiac patients (80%) are at low risk.
- All therapeutic options (subject to specific contraindications) do not increase risk.
- High-risk patients after cardiac therapy may be restratified to low risk and offered ED therapy.

6 Drug therapy

The treatment of ED and the awareness of its frequency and importance stem directly from the introduction of the oral phosphodiesterase type 5 (PDE5) inhibitor sildenafil (Viagra®).

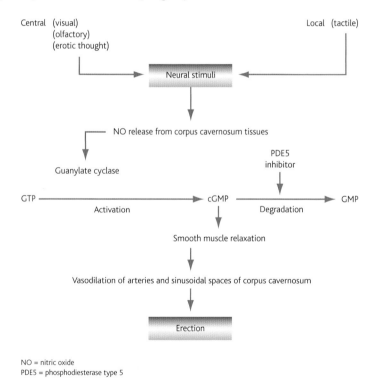

NO = nitric oxide
PDE5 = phosphodiesterase type 5

Figure 6.1 Mode of action of PDE5 inhibitor.

Phosphodiesterase type 5 inhibitors[22]

To say that sildenafil has transformed the management of ED would be a substantial understatement. Its mechanism of action by blocking PDE5's degradation of cGMP promotes blood flow into the penis (see Figure 3.2, page 9) and the restoration of erectile function. Vardenafil and tadalafil have recently been added to this family of drugs. Because their mechanism of action is the same, there is no reason to assume there will be any significant differences in ED effectiveness; however, their PDE selectivity and half-life may be of clinical importance. Potency is not clinically relevant, because it is a way of expressing in vitro concentrations of a drug – in short, given in dose equivalents the clinical end-point will be the same.

Haemodynamically, PDE5 inhibitors have mild nitrate-like actions (sildenafil was originally intended to be a drug for mild angina). As PDE5 is present in smooth muscle cells throughout the vasculature and the NO/cGMP pathway is involved in the regulation of blood pressure, PDE5 inhibitors have a modest hypotensive action. In healthy subjects, a single dose of 100 mg sildenafil transiently lowered blood pressure by an average of 10/7 mmHg, with a return to baseline 6 hours post-dose. There was no effect on heart rate.[23]

As NO is an important neurotransmitter throughout the vasculature and is involved in the regulation of vascular smooth muscle relaxation, a synergistic and clinically important interaction with oral and sublingual nitrates can occur (Appendix 3). A profound fall in blood pressure can result. The mechanism involves the combination of nitrates increasing cGMP formation by activating guanylate cyclase and PDE5 inhibition decreasing cGMP breakdown by inhibiting PDE5. The concomitant administration of PDE5 inhibitors and nitrates is a contraindication to their use and this recommendation also extends to other NO donors such as nicorandil. Clinical guidelines regarding timing of nitrate use post-PDE5 inhibitor or use of a PDE5 inhibitor after cessation of oral or sublingual nitrates are not available, but recent studies are helpful. In a study involving healthy volunteers at 100 mg dosage, sildenafil, with its short half-life (see later), did not react with sublingual nitrates 6 hours post-use. Tadalafil, with it long half-life, did not react at 48 hours. No data are available for vardenafil, but as its half-life is similar to sildenafil, a similar result is to be expected. Oral nitrates are not prognostically important drugs, so they can be discontinued and, if needed, alternative agents substituted. After oral nitrate cessation, and provided there has been no clinical deterioration, PDE5 inhibitors can be used safely. It is recommended that the time interval prior to PDE5 inhibitor use is 5 half-lives, which equals 5 days for the most popular once-daily oral nitrate agents.

When comparing the three PDE5 inhibitors (Figure 6.2), differences are detected in PDE selectivity and half-life.[22] PDEs are functionally heterogeneous enzymes that belong to at least 11 families and comprise at least 45 distinct proteins encoded by at least 21 genes (Table 6.1). Of the reactions studied to date (besides PDE5), the role of PDE6 in visual transduction is the most relevant to clinical practice, since PDE3 is not influenced (potentially an adverse reaction on cardiac myocytes). Tadalafil is 780 times more selective for PDE5 than for PDE6, whereas sildenafil is 6.8 times and vardenafil 2.9 times more selective. Transient visual disturbances, usually a blue haze, are less likely with tadalafil. Tadalafil is, however, an inhibitor of PDE11, which is present in heart, testes, pituitary and prostate tissue. The long-term clinical significance of inhibiting PDE11 is unknown.

Tadalafil has a half-life of 17.5 hours with a period of responsiveness of 36 hours or longer, whereas sildenafil and vardenafil have durations of action

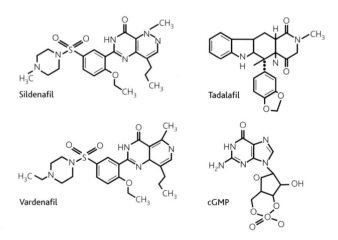

Figure 6.2 Chemical structures of PDE5 inhibitors vs cGMP.

Table 6.1 *Relative selectivity of phosphodiesterase type 5 inhibitors*

Family	Tadalafil	Sildenafil	Vardenafil
PDE1a	20,000	290	630
PDE1b	21,000	1,100	5,000
PDE1c	11,000	110	460
PDE2a	49,000	19,000	72,000
PDE3a	38,000	12,000	7,700
PDE3b	18,000	17,000	15,000
PDE4a	30,000	6,000	46,000
PDE4b	22,000	5,800	33,000
PDE4c	23,000	5,200	34,000
PDE4d	13,000	3,600	16,000
PDE6	780	6.8	2.9
PDE7a	47,000	22,000	200,000
PDE8a	30,000	19,000	310,000
PDE9a	19,000	540	3,600
PDE10a	9,000	3,100	12,000
PDE11a	14	1,500	640

of 3–5 hours. Onset of action following sexual stimulation is approximately 30 minutes, with maximal effect achieved at 1 hour with sildenafil and vardenafil, and 1–2 hours with tadalafil. Tadalafil's absorption is not influenced by food, whereas sildenafil and vardenafil are affected by a fatty meal due to delayed gastric emptying and are more effective 2 hours after food intake.

Sildenafil[24]

Sildenafil is the first oral treatment for ED and the most extensively evaluated. Overall success rates in cardiac patients of ≥80% have been recorded with no evidence of tolerance (decreasing effect over time). Diabetic patients with more complex and extensive pathophysiology have an average success rate of 60% with or without additional risk factors. To date in randomized trials, open-label or outpatient monitoring studies, the use of sildenafil is not associated with any excess risk of myocardial infarction, stroke or mortality. In patients with stable angina, there is no evidence of an ischaemic effect due to coronary steal. In one large exercise study, compared with double-blind placebo, sildenafil 100 mg increased exercise time and diminished ischaemia (Figure 6.3). A study of haemodynamic effects in men with severe CAD identified no adverse cardiovascular effects and a potentially beneficial effect on coronary blood flow reserve.[25] Studies in diabetic and non-diabetic patients have demonstrated improved endothelial function both acutely and after chronic oral dosing, which may have implications beyond the treatment of ED.[23] Sildenafil has also been shown to attenuate the activation of platelet 11b/111a receptor activity. Hypertensive patients on mono- or multiple therapy have experienced no increase in adverse events, with the exception of patients on doxazosin, a non-selec-

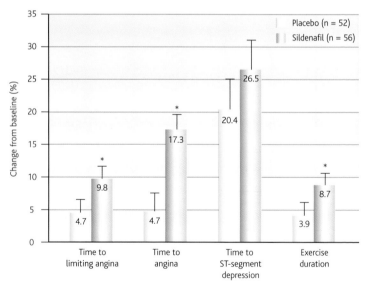

*p<0.05

Figure 6.3 PDE5 inhibition: effects on exercise parameters. (*Source:* Fox KM *et al. Eur Heart J* 2003; **24**: 2206–12)

tive alpha-blocker. Occasional postural effects have occurred when sildenafil was taken within 4 hours of doxazosin 4 mg, so an advisory to avoid this time interval is now in place. Sildenafil has also been proven effective in heart failure patients who were deemed unsuitable for ED therapy (Figure 6.4). The incidence of ED in heart failure subjects is 80%, so this finding is of major clinical importance. Sildenafil dose is on average 50 mg, with 25 mg advised initially in patients older than 80 years, owing to delayed excretion. The 100 mg dose is inevitably needed in diabetic patients. There are several clinical points that need emphasizing:

- The first dose may not be effective and it may take 7–8 attempts before sex is possible. The longer the ED has been a problem and the more severe the ED, the longer for the treatment to reach effectiveness. The patient must be informed of this possibility, or emotional distress can follow the first failure. Very probably this is related to the patient and his partner needing time to become accustomed to having sex again.
- Sexual stimulation is essential.
- An empty stomach, avoiding alcohol or cigarette smoking facilitates the effect.

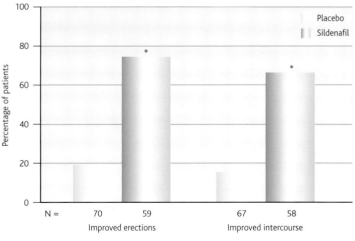

*p<0.0001

Figure 6.4 Sildenafil in patients with CHF: global efficacy assessments at week 12.

- The time to peak effect is approximately 1 hour, with a duration of up to 6 hours.
- The 100 mg dose has no additional adverse cardiac effects above the 50 mg dose and should be routinely prescribed if the 50 mg dose is not effective after 4 attempts.

Sildenafil's short half-life makes it the drug of choice in the more severe cardiac patients, allowing early use of support therapy if an adverse clinical event occurs. Its quick onset of action and predictable duration suit many patients; nonetheless, some couples do complain of a lack of spontaneity – most often the partner.

Tadalafil[26]

Tadalafil has also been extensively evaluated in cardiac patients and has a similar safety and efficacy profile to sildenafil (Figure 6.5). Studies have shown no adverse effects on cardiac contraction, ventricular repolarization or ischaemic threshold. A similar hypotensive effect has been recorded

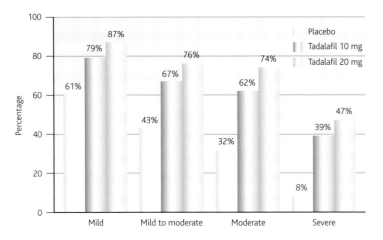

*Positive response to SEP Question 3: 'Did your erection last long enough to have successful intercourse?' ED severity was classified using baseline IIEF EF domain scores as follows: severe (1–10), moderate (11–16), mild to moderate (17–21), mild (22–25), normal (26–30)

Figure 6.5 Percentage of successful intercourse attempts* per group by ED severity.

with doxazosin using 8 mg dosage, so caution is needed. As hypotension does not occur in the supine position and as tadalafil has a long half-life, it is suggested that tadalafil be taken in the morning and doxazosin in the evening. There is no interaction with the selective alpha-blocker tamsulosin, which can therefore be prescribed as an alternative to doxazosin for benign prostatic hypertrophy. Specific recommendations for tadalafil (dose 10 mg and 20 mg) are similar to sildenafil, apart from:

- Food does not affect the onset of activity. However, sexual activity should be avoided within 2 hours of a heavy meal, since it would be occurring at the time of increased cardiac work to digest the food.
- Its peak effect is 1–2 hours.
- Its effective duration has been recorded beyond 36 hours.
- Sublingual nitrates cannot be used for 48 hours post-dose.

Because of its long half-life, tadalafil may not be the first choice for the more complex cardiac cases. However, as 80% of cardiac cases stratify into low risk, it is an alternative for the majority. When spontaneity is an issue, tadalafil is a logical alternative to sildenafil.

Vardenafil[27]

From the very similar structure to sildenafil (see Figure 6.2, page 26), it is not surprising that vardenafil has a similar clinical profile. One study has reported no impairment of exercise ability in stable CAD patients at 10 mg dosage.[28] Similar clinical efficacy for all three agents has been observed in diabetic patients (Figure 6.6).[13] While vardenafil is an alternative to sildenafil, it appears to offer little, if any, therapeutic difference and currently lacks the extensive data supporting the effectiveness and safety of sildenafil and tadalafil. However, there is no reason to assume it is less safe.

Side-effects

As PDE5 inhibitors have the same vasodilating properties, side-effects are similar. Headaches and flushing are the most frequent and are usually well tolerated. Dyspepsia and rhinitis occasionally occur. Adverse event discon-

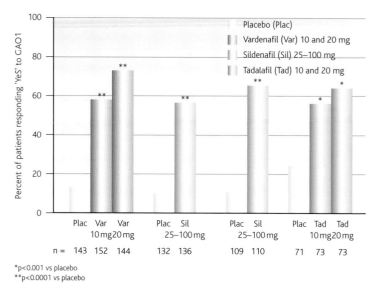

*p<0.001 vs placebo
**p<0.0001 vs placebo

Figure 6.6 Affirmative responses to a global assessment question on improved erections in 4 placebo-controlled, 12-week trials of vardenafil, sildenafil and taladafil in diabetic patients with erectile dysfunction.[13]

tinuation rates are 1% or less. Tadalafil is associated with back pain, which may be due to venous congestion, and affects 5–6%.

Apomorphine[29]

Apomorphine is a D_1/D_2 dopamine-receptor agonist acting specifically in the paraventricular and supraoptic nuclei of the hypothalamus. The subsequent triggering of neural outflow stimulates the spinal cord and parasympathetic outflow increases, leading to smooth muscle relaxation. It is administered sublingually in 2 mg or 3 mg dosages, acting rapidly. Its peak effect occurs in 15–20 minutes, allowing a rapid response if sexual activity begins. Its overall efficacy is less than the PDE5 inhibitors and is confined to the milder cases of ED. Compared with placebo in non-diabetic patients, the percentage of attempts resulting in an erection firm enough for sexual

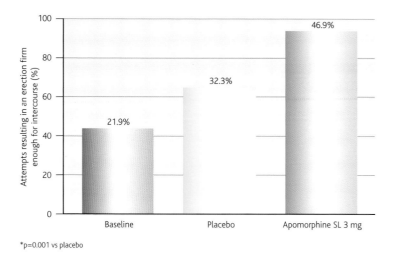

*p=0.001 vs placebo

Figure 6.7 Apomorphine SL (3 mg): percentage of attempts with erection firm enough for intercourse. (*Source:* Dula E *et al. Eur Urol* 2001; **39**: 558–64)

intercourse using 2 mg or 3 mg was 47% versus 34.8% (p<0.001) (Figure 6.7). Safety has been established in patients with hypertension, CAD, hyperlipidaemia, and diabetes. No significant cardiovascular drug interactions have been recorded and concomitant nitrate use is not a contraindication. As it is an emetic, side-effects include nausea (5%); this is dose-related and tends to diminish with repeated drug exposure. Other adverse effects include:

- headache
- dizziness
- somnolence
- syncope (rarely)

In clinical practice the response to apomorphine has been disappointing in comparison with the PDE5 inhibitors and this is almost certainly due to the ED fault being mainly peripheral at the endothelial level rather than central. Nevertheless, in milder cases, it provides an alternative choice which may suit some couples.

Other oral agents

Yohimbine, an alpha-receptor antagonist, is widely available. It acts centrally and peripherally.[30] Properly designed trials have not been performed and its efficacy has not been established. In the era of evidence-based medicine, it cannot be recommended.

Phentolamine has been studied in buccal formulation but is not approved for the treatment of ED. Concerns about the cardiovascular adverse potential will be a significant problem.

L-arginine is the source of NO and is usually present in abundance. L-arginine deficiency, which can occur in hyperlipidaemia, renal patients and some diabetic patients, might respond to supplementation, but no data exist to support this concept.

Key points

- PDE5 inhibitors have transformed the management of ED.
- They are safe in properly assessed cardiac patients.
- Their proper use requires careful explanation to achieve maximal benefit.

Other therapies

7

It is important to emphasize that no therapy increases cardiovascular risk provided that the guidelines are followed (see Table 5.1, pages 20–1) and contraindications observed.[2,31]

Lifestyle

Avoiding cigarette smoking, eating a healthy diet and having regular exercise can all be helpful, not just for the ED but also for the underlying vascular pathology.

Certain bicycle seats can damage the penile circulation and therefore long-distance cycling or mountain biking, may not have the same exercise benefits.

Psychosexual therapy

If psychogenic ED is present (see page 11), appropriate counselling should be arranged. Organic ED will have a psychological component secondary to the ED, but this usually responds to the ED therapy and sildenafil has been documented to help relieve the depression induced by ED. It is not common for psychotherapy and sex therapy to be needed if the ED cause is clearly explained, the man is reassured and not left to feel guilty or 'useless', treatment is encouraged and detailed advice and support given. Nonetheless, psychosexual therapy should not be viewed as a stigma, given its important role in selected cases. Team working is valuable (physician and therapist) where organic and psychological causes overlap. Indeed, fully trained and accredited psychosexual and couple therapists play an important role in the management of ED when the psychogenic component is significant.

Hormonal therapy

Occasionally, male hypogonadism is detected by identifying low levels of testosterone. Pituitary failure should be excluded. Usually, patients report loss of libido (sex drive).

If a random testosterone level is low, then it should be confirmed by a 9 am testosterone level. A decreased luteinizing hormone (LH) suggests a pituitary cause, while increased LH suggests the more common testicular failure.

Proven androgen deficiency can be treated with oral, intramuscular or transdermal testosterone. Regular monitoring with prostate-specific antigen (PSA) measurements every 6 months is advised in view of the risk of prostate cancer in men and its relationship to testosterone.

Vacuum constriction devices

Vacuum constriction devices are a long-established means of treating ED. They are a non-invasive method which produce an erection by removing the air around the penis, as they create a vacuum of up to 250 mmHg. Blood flows into the penis and is held there by using a rubber ring to constrict the base of the penis. The constriction ring must not be left in place longer than 30 minutes, since ischaemic damage may result.

Erections can be successfully achieved in the majority of cases, but the device should only be used when drug therapy has failed or is contraindicated. It is simple and safe, yet its use interrupts foreplay, impairs spontaneity and may produce a cold cyanotic penis. As the penis is flaccid between the ring and the body, it may pivot at its base and feel floppy.

A haematoma (minor in 10% of cases) may occur significantly in men on anticoagulants, so this is a relative contraindication and specific training and advice are needed. Vacuum devices should not be advocated for men with penile curvature.

Injection therapy

Direct intracavernosal injection of several medications began in the 1980s.

Prostaglandin E1 is a natural substance which relaxes smooth muscle cells and dilates the arterioles, increasing blood flow into the penis. Prostaglandin E1 (alprostadil) is licensed for use and is effective in 5–15 minutes with an erection that usually lasts 30 minutes but occasionally several hours. The starting dose is 1.25 μg and can be increased to 20 μg, depending on effect. On removal of the needle, firm pressure is applied and the drug gently massaged into the penis for 30 seconds or so. Some men find walking up and down stimulates penile blood flow. Men on anticoagulants should press for 5–10 minutes.

The erection occurs without stimulation, though stimulation may enhance its effects. It is important that patients are taught the correct technique. The erections are occasionally painful but usually feel natural. It is recommended that this treatment not be used more frequently than every 4 days.

Alprostadil is effective in up to 80% of cases and is associated with a return to spontaneous erections in 35%. It is safe and effective in diabetic patients who are used to self-injection if on insulin. Partners often inject as part of the sexual activity.

Though effective, the discontinuation rate is high – local pain and loss of spontaneity are the most common reasons. Contraindications are few and include:

- haematological problems (leukaemia, sickle cell disease, and risk of priapism)
- schizophrenia
- Peyronie's disease

Side-effects are not common: infection, bleeding and bruising suggest poor technique, and flushing from vasodilation. Hypotension is rare. Repeated injections at the same site can cause fibrosis, leading to impaired erection and penile curvature.

The only serious short-term side-effect is priapism. All patients should be issued with information on how to manage this. If the erection lasts over 4 hours and is not reduced by vigorous walking or being wrapped in a bag of frozen peas or crushed ice, the corpora will need aspirating.

Men with poor dexterity (e.g. arthritic hands or tremor) will need their partner's help with the injection.

Transurethral therapy

Intraurethral therapy of alprostadil is an alternative to injections. Medicated Urethral System for Erection (MUSE) involves inserting a 1.4 mm pellet, using a hand-held applicator, into the urethra about 15 minutes prior to sex. After micturition, a dose of 125 μg, 250 μg, 500 μg or 1000 μg is deployed – much higher than injection therapy owing to drug loss in the general circulation. Two doses are allowed per 24 hours.

Once the correct dose has been identified, success rates of up to 60% have been recorded, though in a comparative study with injections this fell to 43% (injections, 70%).

Side-effects include:

- urethral pain or irritation (up to 30%)
- dizziness
- perspiration
- hypotension

Females sometimes complain of vaginal discomfort. In addition, as prostaglandin E1 can induce labour, a condom should be used if pregnancy is suspected or established.

Erections usually last 30–60 minutes and priapism is rare.

Surgical treatment

When all else fails or when there is a history of trauma, penile surgery offers another therapeutic route. Once more, cardiac patients should be offered surgery rather than be denied this option. Clearly, specialist referral and advice is needed and referral to the urologist is advised, with the cardiologist outlining risk from the cardiac perspective.

Surgery may be vascular (ligature of venous incompetence or arterial revascularization) or involve penile prosthetic surgery. Patient satisfaction with penile prostheses ranges from 66–92% (partners, 60–80%).

Key points

- Oral therapy is the preferred option.
- Injection or transurethral therapy is safe and effective.
- Vacuum devices also are an effective alternative, though care and special training are needed if the patient is on warfarin.
- Surgery is seldom needed but should not be denied to cardiac patients.
- Cardiac patients have sexual needs which must be addressed.

Specific cardiac conditions and sex[2]

Use the Sexual Health Inventory for Men (SHIM) which is the shortened version of the IIEF (see Table 5.2, page 22) and reproduced in the Appendix (see page 59). Check the level of daily activity compared with the level of exertion during sex using the METs guide (see page 2). Use exercise electrocardiography if unsure or echocardiography to clarify valve status or left ventricular function. Always try to involve the partner in the ED advice programme – although ED is a man's problem, it is a couple's concern.

Hypertension

- This is not a contraindication to sex when controlled.
- Controlled patients: antihypertensives (single or multiple) are not a contraindication, but use caution with doxazosin (and therefore all alpha-blockers that are non-selective) and PDE5 inhibitors.
- All ED therapies can be utilized.
- Antihypertensives least likely to cause ED are the angiotensin II receptor antagonists and doxazosin.

Angina

- For stable patients, there is minimal risk for sex or ED therapy.
- Nitrates and nicorandil are contraindications to PDE5 inhibitors. On most occasions these can safely be discontinued.
- Heart rate-slowing drugs are the most effective anti-anginal agents: beta-blockers, verapamil, diltiazem.
- Use an exercise ECG to stratify risk (see page 2), if unsure.

Postmyocardial infarction

▥ Use pre- or postdischarge exercise ECG to guide advice; no need for delay to sex resumption if satisfactory.

▥ Advise gentle return to allow for losses of confidence by both patient and partner.

▥ Rehabilitation programmes are a positive advantage.

▥ Avoid sex in first 2 weeks (period of maximal risk).

Post-surgery or percutaneous intervention

▥ If successful, risk is low.

▥ Sternal scar may be painful; advise side-to-side position or patient on top position.

▥ Male chest hairs grow back like bristle; advise small pillow between partners to avoid the pain.

▥ Use exercise ECG, if unsure of ability.

Cardiac failure

▥ The risk is low, if good ability.

▥ If symptomatic, adjust medication accordingly; patient may need to be the more passive partner.

▥ If severely symptomatic, sex may not be possible owing to physical limitations and can occasionally trigger decompensation.

▥ An exercise programme can facilitate the return to sex; physically fit equals sexually fit.

Valve disease

▥ For mild cases, there is no increased risk.

▥ Antibiotic prophylaxis is not needed.

▥ Significant aortic stenosis may lead to sudden death and can be worsened by the vasodilatory effects of PDE5 inhibitors.

Arrhythmias

▓ Controlled atrial fibrillation is not an increased risk depending on cause and exercise ability.
▓ Warfarin contraindicates vacuum device and requires caution with injections.
▓ Complex arrhythmias: arrange for 24–48 hour ambulatory ECG monitoring and exercise testing. Treat and retest
▓ Pacemakers are not a contraindication.
▓ With implanted defibrillators, use exercise test for safety before advising. This is usually not a problem.

Other conditions

▓ For pericarditis, await full recovery; there is no specific increased risk thereafter.
▓ With peripheral vascular disease, stroke or transient ischaemic attacks (TIAs), there is increased risk of myocardial infarct, therefore screen.
▓ With hypertrophic obstructive cardiomyopathy, there is increased risk of syncope and sudden death on exercise. Exercise ECG advised. PDE5 and alprostadil may increase the degree of obstruction owing to vasodilatory effects. Test dose under hospital supervision is recommended.

An assessment algorithm (Figure 8.1, page 44) summarizes management guidelines.

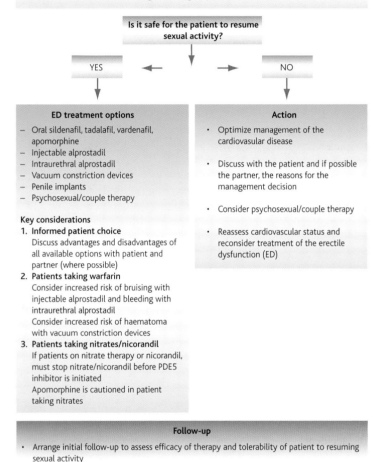

ASSESSMENT
- Consider level of normal daily activities compared with the level of exertion associated with resuming sexual activity
- Conduct routine ED investigations
- Grade as low, intermediate or high risk using simple criteria in Table 5.1

Is it safe for the patient to resume sexual activity?

YES ← → NO

ED treatment options
- Oral sildenafil, tadalafil, vardenafil, apomorphine
- Injectable alprostadil
- Intraurethral alprostadil
- Vacuum constriction devices
- Penile implants
- Psychosexual/couple therapy

Key considerations
1. **Informed patient choice**
   Discuss advantages and disadvantages of all available options with patient and partner (where possible)
2. **Patients taking warfarin**
   Consider increased risk of bruising with injectable alprostadil and bleeding with intraurethral alprostadil
   Consider increased risk of haematoma with vacuum constriction devices
3. **Patients taking nitrates/nicorandil**
   If patients on nitrate therapy or nicorandil, must stop nitrate/nicorandil before PDE5 inhibitor is initiated
   Apomorphine is cautioned in patient taking nitrates

Action
- Optimize management of the cardiovasular disease
- Discuss with the patient and if possible the partner, the reasons for the management decision
- Consider psychosexual/couple therapy
- Reassess cardiovascular status and reconsider treatment of the erectile dysfunction (ED)

Follow-up
- Arrange initial follow-up to assess efficacy of therapy and tolerability of patient to resuming sexual activity
- After initital follow-up, ED assessments can be conducted as routine checks for cardiovascular symptoms. Discuss compliance and any recurrence of spontaneous erections

Figure 8.1 Management algorithm of erectile dysfunction with diagnosed cardio-vascular disease.

Stroke

9

Stroke is a difficult and sensitive area for the victim and partner. Minimal disability from a transient ischaemic attack (TIA) has been mentioned (see page 43) and here the main focus is looking for additional cardiovascular risk and minimizing it. Sex should not present a management problem and the couple can be reassured about the minimal risk of a further stroke with modern management (e.g. statin, ACE inhibitor, aspirin).

Where physical appearance is a problem, then open discussion is essential and sexual counselling may be needed. Strokes are often followed by fatigue and a decreased libido, as well as depression, and ED may be the consequence. Depression is very common after a stroke but may well respond to specific therapy.

Those sexually active before a stroke are the most likely to be active again; nevertheless, it takes time and support. Touching, kissing and caressing are good starting contacts. As fatigue is often a problem, suggest the morning time after a good night's sleep.

Stroke patients with a urinary catheter can be advised to remove it for the sexual activity and insert it after. Avoiding fluids for 2 hours before sex will decrease the bladder volume. If the catheter cannot be removed, it can be folded back over the erect penis and covered with a prelubricated condom. Women victims of stroke can tape the catheter to the abdomen or thigh. Tell the patients to open their bowels before sex to avoid any embarrassing accidents.

Paralysis

Paralysis will inevitably lead to the need to change the person's usual position. As positions (within the bounds of common sense!) do not increase cardiac stress, experimentation is going to be necessary. Pillows can be used to offer support in the side-to-side position.

The most common positions that stroke victims find most useful are:

▦ Stroke victim lies on back, partner on top.
▦ Side-to-side position. Stroke victim lies on affected side with pillows to support (back and hips).
▦ Sitting position (male victim) in wheelchair or on a sofa or chair.

As stroke victims can lose sensation, advise the partner to make contact with the non-affected side. If speech is a problem or comprehension, visual communication and touch are ways of expressing feelings.

Self-stimulation, mutual masturbation and oral sex are other alternatives. Female lubrication problems can be helped with water-soluble lubricants (e.g. KY jelly).

Finally, always be supportive to the couple and try to keep them away from performance issues using lots of humour because they will experience failure where they did not before. This must be anticipated and not allowed to become an overwhelming issue.

Key points
▦ Stroke victims can resume sex but will need specialized advice.
▦ ED can be treated and there are no specific contraindications.

Female sexual dysfunction

10

From the cardiac viewpoint, sex is the same for both men and women.[2] Female sexual problems may occur as a consequence of cardiac illness or drug therapy.

Women may experience a reduction in desire, a lack of ability to orgasm, lubrication problems leading to pain on intercourse and vaginismus.

Female sexual dysfunction is a significant problem with no specific treatment, though research continues with the PDE5 inhibitors and apomorphine.

Antidepressants (especially the SSRIs) and beta blockers can reduce libido and diuretics can cause lubrication difficulties. Therapeutic changes may, therefore, be helpful and lubricants are widely available.

When treating a man's ED, it is important to remember the female partner who may need advice beyond the usual given to the couple.

After experiencing a cardiac event or stroke, women should receive the same advice as men on returning to sexual activity.

For a detailed overview of management, a chapter by Munarriz and colleagues in *Hot Topics in Urology* is recommended reading (see page 55).

Follow-up

It is important to follow up all men with ED and an appointment 4 weeks after advising on treatment is recommended.

- Is the oral treatment working?
- Is the oral treatment being used properly?
- Is the dose correct?
- Are the couple happy with the treatment?
- If using injections, are there any problems?
- Is the vacuum device satisfactory?

Remember always to tell the patient the first dose of a PDE5 inhibitor may not be effective and it may take 7 or 8 attempts before it 'kicks in'. Use the analogy of reconditioning an engine.

Referral

Not everyone wants to treat ED or advise on sex. If it is not your 'cup of tea' – refer. In a primary care practice try to establish a policy either doctor- or nurse-led. If specialist help is required, refer to the urologist/physician/diabetologist/cardiologist who has a special interest. Never give up: sex is too important to the relationship.

Often a nurse is the best person to advise and, from my experience, the most successful. Patients volunteering their ED have often required considerable courage to do so, so always give them the time; if you do not have time, call them back for a dedicated appointment. ED may be mentioned at the end of a consultation, 'By the way ...' or as the patient is leaving – 'the door knob syndrome'. Don't ignore the effort it took.

13 The cardiovascular potential of PDE5 inhibitors

As PDE5 inhibitors are in effect vasodilators, they may have an important therapeutic role when vasoconstriction is clinically important. Research progresses in hypertension, cardiac failure and Raynaud's phenomenon.[32,33]

The therapeutic potential is exciting, given the reports of major benefits in treating pulmonary hypertension.[34]

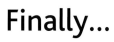

Finally...

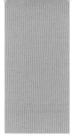

Please feel free to copy or use any of this book if you think it will help in the management of your patients. A note of acknowledgement would be welcome. Oh, and if this book should run to more editions, ideas and suggestions will be acted on. I have now supervised a male cardiovascular sexual health clinic for over 3 years with my nurse Emma Martin: it is one of the most rewarding initiatives that I have undertaken. Sex, the heart and ED is an important issue for many couples – most can be helped so give it a try (or refer).

Further information

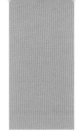

The British Journal of Diabetes and Vascular Disease July/Aug 2002. Vol. 2, issue 4.

Eardley I, Sethia K. *Erectile Dysfunction: Current investigations and management*. 2nd edition. London: Mosby, 2003.

Kirby M. *Erectile Dysfunction and Vascular Disease*. Oxford: Blackwell Publishing, 2003.

Kirby RS, O'Leary MP, eds. *Hot Topics in Urology*. London: Saunders, 2004.

Sexual Dysfunction Association = *www.SDA.uk.net*

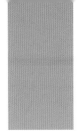

References

1. Drory Y. Sexual activity and cardiovascular risk. *Eur Heart J Supplement* 2002; **4**(suppl H): H13–H18.

2. Jackson G, Betteridge J, Dean J *et al.* A systematic approach to erectile dysfunction in the cardiovascular patient: a consensus statement – update 2002. *Int J Clin Pract* 2002; **56**: 633–71.

3. Müller JE, Mittleman A, MacLure M *et al.* Determinants of myocardial infarction onset study investigators. Triggering myocardial infarction by sexual activity: low absolute risk and prevention by regular physical exercise. *JAMA* 1996; **275**: 1405–9.

4. Müller J, Ahlbom A, Hulting J *et al.* Sexual activity as a trigger of myocardial infarction: a case cross-over analysis in the Stockholm Heart Epidemiology Programme (SHEEP). *Heart* 2001; **86**: 387–90.

5. NIH Consensus Conference. Impotence. NIH Consensus Development Panel on Impotence. *JAMA* 1993; **270**: 83–90.

6. Ayta IA, McKinlay JB, Krane RJ. The likely worldwide increase in erectile dysfunction between 1995 and 2025 and some possible policy consequences. *BJU Int* 1999; **84**: 50–6.

7. Impotence Association Survey. *Attitudes towards Erectile Dysfunction*. London: Impotence Association, 2002.

8. Marwick C. Survey says patients expect little physician help on sex. *JAMA* 1999; **281**: 2173–4.

9. Bortolotti A, Parazzini F, Colli E, Landoni M. The epidemiology of erectile dysfunction and its risk factors. *Int J Androl* 1997; **20**: 323–34.

10. Eardley I. Pathophysiology of erectile dysfunction. *Br J Diabetes Vasc Dis* 2002; **2**: 272–6.

11. Feldman HA, Goldstein I, Hatzichristou DG *et al*. Impotence and its medical and psychological correlates: results of the Massachusetts Male Aging Study. *J Urol* 1994; **151**: 54–61.

12. Roumeguère Th, Wespes E, Carpentier Y *et al*. Erectile dysfunction is associated with a high prevalence of hyperlipidaemia and coronary heart disease risk. *Eur Urol* 2003; **44**: 355–9.

13. Snow KJ. Erectile dysfunction in patients with diabetes mellitus – advances in treatment with phosphodiesterase type 5 inhibitors. *Br J Diabetes Vasc Dis* 2002; **2**: 282–7.

14. Solomon H, Man JW, Jackson G. Erectile dysfunction and the cardiac patient: endothelial dysfunction is the common denominator. *Heart* 2003; **89**: 251–4.

15. Kirby M, Jackson G, Betteridge J, Friedli K. Is erectile dysfunction a marker for cardiovascular disease? *Int J Clin Pract* 2001; **55**: 614–18.

16. Pritzker M. The penile stress test: a window to the heart of the man? *Circulation* 1999; **100**: 3751 (abst).

17. Solomon H, Man JW, Wierzbicki AS, Jackson G. Relation of erectile dysfunction to angiographic coronary artery disease. *Am J Cardiol* 2003; **91**: 230–1.

18. Greenstein A, Chen J, Miller H *et al*. Does severity of ischaemic coronary disease correlate with erectile function? *Int J Impot Res* 1997; **9**: 123–6.

19. Solomon H, Man J, Wierzbicki AS *et al*. Erectile dysfunction: cardiovascular risk and the role of the cardiologist. *Int J Clin Pract* 2003; **57**: 96–9.

20. DeBusk R, Drory Y, Goldstein I *et al*. Management of sexual dysfunction in patients with cardiovascular disease: recommendations of the Princeton Consensus Panel. *Am J Cardiol* 2000; **86**: 175–81.

21. Rosen RC, Riley A, Wagner G *et al*. The International Index of Erectile Dysfunction (IIEF): A multidimensional scale for assessment of erectile dysfunction. *Urology* 1997; **49**: 822–30.

22. Giuliano F. Phosphodiesterase type 5 inhibition in erectile dysfunction: an overview. *Eur Heart J Supplements* 2002; **4** (Suppl H): H7–H12.

23. Gillies HC, Roblin D, Jackson G. Coronary and systemic hemodynamic effects of sildenafil citrate: from basic science to clinical studies in patients with cardiovascular disease. *Int J Cardiol* 2002; **86**: 131–41.

24. Padma-Nathan H (editor). Sildenafil citrate (Viagra®) and erectile dysfunction: a comprehensive four year update on efficacy, safety, and management approaches. *Urology* 2002; **60**: 1–90.

25. Herrmann HC, Chang G, Klugherz BD, Mahoney PD. Hemodynamic effects of sildenafil in men with severe coronary artery disease. *N Engl J Med* 2000; **342**: 1662–6.

26. Brock GB, McMahon CG, Chen KK *et al*. Efficiency and safety of tadalafil for the treatment of erectile dysfunction: results of integrated analysis. *J Urol* 2002; **168**: 1332–6.

27. Porst H, Rosen R, Padma-Nathan H *et al*. Efficacy and tolerability of vardenafil, a new selective phosphodiesterase type 5 inhibitor, in patients with erectile dysfunction. The first at home clinical trial. *Int J Impot Res* 2001; **13**: 192–9.

28. Thadani U, Smith W, Nash S *et al*. The effect of vardenafil, a potent and highly selective phosphodiesterase-5 inhibitor for the treatment of erectile dysfunction, on the cardiovascular response to exercise in patients with coronary artery disease. *J Am Coll Cardiol* 2002; **40**: 2006–12.

29. Heaton JPW. Key issues from the clinical trials of apomorphine SL. *World J Urol* 2001; **19**: 25–3.

30. Morales A, Yohimbine in erectile dysfunction: the facts. *Int J Impot Res* 2000; **12** (Suppl 1): 570–74.

31. Ali W, Besarani D, Kirby R. Modern treatment of erectile dysfunction. *Br J Diabetes Vas Dis* 2002; **2**: 255–61.

32. Halcox JPJ, Nour KRA, Zalos G *et al*. The effect of sildenafil on human vascular function, platelet activation and myocardial ischaemia. *J Am Coll Cardiol* 2002; **40**: 1232–40.

33. Katz SD. Potential role of type 5 phosphodiesterase inhibition in the treatment of congestive heart failure. *Congest Heart Fail* 2003; **9**: 9–15.

34. Jackson G. PDE 5 inhibitors: looking beyond ED. *Int J Clin Pract* 2003; **57**: 159–60.

Appendix 1

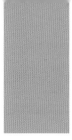

Sexual health inventory for men

Patient's name: . . . . Date of Evaluation: . . . .

Sexual health is an important part of an individual's overall physical and emotional well-being. Erectile dysfunction, also known as impotence, is one type of a very common medical condition affecting sexual health. Fortunately, there are many different treatment options for erectile dysfunction. This questionnaire is designed to help you and your doctor identify if you may be experiencing erectile dysfunction. If you are, you may choose to discuss treatment options with your doctor.

Each question has several possible responses. Circle the number of the response that best describes your own situation. Please be sure that you select one and only one response for each question.

Over the past 6 months:

1. How do you rate your *confidence* that you could get and keep an erection?

Very low	1
Low	2
Moderate	3
High	4
Very high	5

2. When you had erections with sexual stimulation, *how often* were your erections hard enough for penetration (entering your partner)?

No sexual activity	0
Almost never or never	1
A few times (much less than half the time)	2
Sometimes (about half the time)	3
Most times (much more than half the time)	4
Almost always or always	5

3. During sexual intercourse, *how often* were you able to maintain your erection after you had penetrated (entered) your partner?

Did not attempt intercourse	0
Almost never or never	1
A few times (much less than half the time)	2
Sometimes (about half the time)	3
Most times (much more than half the time)	4
Almost always or always	5

4. During sexual intercourse, *how difficult* was it to maintain your erection to completion of intercourse?

Did not attempt intercourse	0
Extremely difficult	1
Very difficult	2
Difficult	3
Slightly difficult	4
Not difficult	5

5. When you attempted sexual intercourse, *how often* was it satisfactory for you?

Did not attempt intercourse	0
Almost never or never	1
A few times (much less than half the time)	2
Sometimes (about half the time)	3
Most times (much more than half the time)	4
Almost always or always	5

Add the numbers corresponding to questions 1–5. If you score is 21 or less, you may be showing signs of erectile dysfunction and may want to speak with your doctor.

Score . . . .

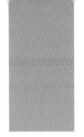

Appendix 2

Routine clinical investigations for erectile dysfunction

The routine clinical investigations for ED should also be carried out in the cardiovascular patient experiencing erectile problems, namely:

- physical examination of the penis and testes
- blood pressure measurement
- fasting lipid profile and blood glucose

For patients with a loss of libido (sexual drive), consider:

- random testosterone level – to screen for hypogonadism. If testosterone levels are low, measurment of HBG, FSH/LH and/or prolactin levels will help to identify the most likely cause.

Further investigations should be considered based upon the findings from the patient's history and examinations. When there is doubt over the cardiovascular risk in a patient returning to sexual activity, consider:

- simple exercise test – as an approximate guide to equivalent exercise tolerance, refer to METs Table 1.1, page 2)
- exercise ECG

Appendix 3

Common nitrate preparations

Glyceryl trinitrate	Isosorbide dinitrate	Isosorbide mononitrate
Coro-Nitro pump spray	Angitak	Elantan
Glytrin spray	Isordil	Ismo
GTN 300 µg	Sorbichew	Isotrate
Nitrolingual spray pump	Sorbitrate	Monit
Nitromin	Cedocard Retard	Mono-Cedocard
Suscard	Isoket Retard	Chemydur 60XL
Sustac	Isordil Tembids	Elantan
	Sorbid SA	Imdur
Transdermal preparations	Isoket	Isib 60XL
Deponit		Ismo Retard
Minitran	*Transdermal*	Isotard
Nitro-Dur	*preparation*	MCR-50
Percutol	Isocard	Modisal XL
Transderm-Nitro		Monit SR
		Monomax SR
		Monosorb XL 60

- Patients may not know they are on nitrate therapy, so it is important to mention trade names or, better still, ask the patient to bring his medication to the consultation

- Discussion about nitrates should always include mention of 'poppers' (amyl nitrate)

Appendix 4

Grading of angina by effort by the Canadian Cardiovascular Society

Minimal/'mild' angina

1. 'Ordinary physical activity does not cause angina': this includes walking and climbing stairs. Angina with strenuous or rapid or prolonged exertion at work or recreation.

2. 'Slight limitation of ordinary activity': this includes walking or climbing stairs rapidly, walking uphill, walking or stair-climbing after meals, or in cold, or in wind, or under emotional stress, or only during the few hours after awakening; walking more than two blocks[*] on the level and climbing more than one flight of ordinary stairs at a normal pace and in normal conditions.

'Moderate' angina

3. 'Marked limitation of ordinary physical activity'; this includes walking one to two blocks[*] on the level and climbing one flight of stairs in normal conditions and at normal pace.

'Severe' angina

4. 'Inability to carry on any physical activity without discomfort – anginal syndrome may be present at rest'.

[*]100 metres/yards

Appendix 5

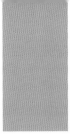

New York Heart Association classification of congestive heart failure

Class I   Patients with cardiac disease but with no limitation during ordinary physical activity

Class II   Slight limitations caused by cardiac disease. Activity such as walking causes dyspnoea

Class III Marked limitation; symptoms are provoked easily, e.g. by walking on the flat

Class IV   Breathlessness at rest

Index